Lives
Touched
by
Down Syndrome

Thank you contributors to this book. Thank you for writing your story and for your willingness to share how your life is touched by Down syndrome.

Thank you Janci Patterson for assisting in editing this book.

ISBN: 978-1-4116-6405-0

Printed in the U.S.A.

Table of Contents

Introduction

When Jeffrey joined our family I felt like we were admitted to a special club. Suddenly people were visiting us who had children with Down syndrome. The general theme of these visits or calls was, "Welcome to the adventure!"

From the moment Jeffrey was born people started sharing their stories with us. I remember one father bringing presents for Jeffrey and telling us about his son, Seth. Seth had just recently said "Mama" for the first time and really knew what he was saying. Seth's father tearfully shared how exciting this was because it had taken eighteen months to reach this moment.

After hearing and being touched by so many stories I decided to collect them in a book for others to enjoy. They are treasures. No matter what stage a person is at in the lifelong adventure of knowing someone with Down syndrome, he or she will find something to relate to or laugh with in this book.

For the many parents who find out they are having a child with Down syndrome and do not know what to expect, this book provides something more personal than a scientific and general study of Down syndrome. This book is made up of experiences about what life is like knowing someone with Down syndrome.

These stories range in theme from comical to inspirational. Many of the stories reflect the influence of the author's religious beliefs.

These stories come from across the United States and Canada. They are written by parents, grandparents, teachers and friends. And they are all about lives touched by Down syndrome.

Enjoy!

Justin

Justin, at thirteen, is our oldest child with Down syndrome. He loves to watch movies, especially Disney animated features and musical children's programs. He will watch his favorites so many times that he can (and always does) repeat the lines of the movie and sing the songs right along with the characters.

A few years ago, Justin's favorite movie was *The Lion King*. We didn't realize how much he thought about this movie until one day when he exhibited the most puzzling behavior. He spent a considerable amount of time outside, catching our somewhat antisocial cat, Goliath. He would bring the cat inside, where he would climb onto the piano bench that he had placed in the middle of the living room floor. There Justin would stand and hold our poor, scared, orange cat way up high, with Goliath's kitty legs just hanging there in front of Justin's face.

Justin did this a number of times that day, until we were certain that poor Goliath would run away from home the next time he got away. Yet, somehow, Justin managed to catch Goliath yet again and climb that piano bench, displaying Goliath for all to see. At this point our daughter Heather walked into the room and said, "Mom , that's funny. Justin looks just like Rafiki, that monkey in *The Lion King*. And Goliath looks just like Simba, hanging there like that!" We laughed so hard when we realized that all day long, Justin had been re-enacting his favorite scene from *The Lion King*!

Janet McClellan

Liza

Liza asks for a hamburger daily. Everyone who knows her has heard her mention this favorite food. Due to nutritional concerns, her polite requests aren't met as often as she would like. But, each time she asks I smile for many reasons.

The past six years have been filled with worry, struggles, love and laughter. I can no longer remember myself without the challenge and joy Liza has brought to my life. When Liza was four months old, she had surgery to repair a hole in her heart. Prior to her surgery, she was too exhausted and weak to eat. Liza did not gain weight, so life became overwhelming with endless doctor visits and feeding therapy sessions. She was only nine pounds at the time of her surgery, lighter than we had hoped.

Following her surgery, the low muscle tone in her mouth made it difficult for Liza to eat many solids. As a toddler, she kept meat and many other tough foods in her mouth for a long time, but couldn't swallow them. We were living in Japan and didn't have much help. We even flew back to the United States to see a feeding team consisting of doctors and therapists. While we didn't find many immediate answers, Liza made progress and the feeding issue slowly cleared up.

During all this time, Liza attended physical therapy, occupational therapy and speech weekly. She began walking at 30 months. We cheered with her as her vocabulary grew. We quickly learned that Liza was good at applauding her own successes. She has become personable and confident.

Last year, when I attended the open house for Liza's dance class, I laughed and cried as I realized how far she had come. She not only followed every dance step, but she waved "hi Mom" and said, "hamburger lunch...with cheese...oh, and ketchup," at the same time she was tapping to the music. Now I don't have to worry about Liza's ability to eat because she can polish off a hamburger quicker than anyone in our family and she enjoys every bite.

Carol Truncellito

Lorren

From the moment she was born our Lorren was a fighter. Not only did she have Down syndrome, but her stomach and intestines were not connected.

When we finally saw our grandchild after her surgery my first impression was of a baby being tortured with needles. I had to overcome my fear of hurting her when the nurse suggested that I hold her. Here the magic started. One of my tears fell on her face and she looked up and smiled. I was mesmerized! From then on she and I have had an unbelievable relationship.

Since Lorren reached school age she has spent every other weekend with us. She comes with a suitcase, a bag of favorite videos and cosmetic case, usually packed well ahead of time in anticipation.

Lorren has a way of saying the most unexpected things at the most opportune times. We call these phrases "Lorrenisms."

At Christmas-time I was taking breakfast orders, trying to be a short order cook. Lorren waited patiently, then asked, "How about me?" Her order: "fo ba." After being asked for the third time she put hands on hips and glared. "I'm not going to tell you again!" She got down from her chair, dragged me to the pantry and pointed, "There." Of course, Fruit Bar!

Most of the time when Lorren speaks I can figure out what she's saying. But one time she kept repeating what I thought was "p-plan." Finally, she went to my scarf drawer, put a scarf around her neck and with arms akimbo said, "I can fly…" Of course, Peter Pan!

Another time, my sister and a niece invited Lorren and me to go for a ride in her car. It was suggested that we play the alphabet game, taking turns naming an animal that started with the next letter of the alphabet. Lorren went first. She said, "Apple." We protested that an apple wasn't an animal. She thought a moment and said, "I know. Apple worm."

The most precious Lorrenism occurred when she awakened me, her little nose touching mine and said, "Grammer, you are my best friend."

We are lucky to have such a grandchild.

Grammer and Papa Kneisel

Laura

Laura struggled academically and I was concerned about it until her former Early Intervention teacher said, "Don't worry about it. Stress the importance of good social skills. If Laura learns to get along well with others, people won't care that she can't read. On the other hand, if Laura can read but has poor social skills, they won't care about her at all."

I pondered that advice and realized it had truth in it. I didn't give up on teaching her learning skills, but my focus was now on social behavior. I gave her as many social experiences as I could. I proudly and lovingly raised her in the same way I raised my other children.

With the help of her sister, brothers, friends and teachers, Laura developed her social skills and was well liked. Friends became very important to Laura and they had no idea the impact their small acts of kindness had on her. She grew to be a lovely young lady with a friendly, bubbly personality and a great sense of humor. Her radiant smile made her glow from within.

In high school Laura watched the cheerleaders with admiration and was determined that she would be a cheerleader too. She stood by the sidelines of the games and learned each move the girls made. She cheered right along with them and was soon made an honorary cheerleader.

With tremendous enthusiasm, she cheered at each home football and basketball game and the crowd joined in with her. Many people came to the games just to watch her cheer. She was later honored at an assembly for being the student with the most school spirit and was awarded an official, personalized cheerleading jacket. A local sportswriter wrote an article about how much he was inspired by her courage and determination.

I knew she had great friends and was happy at school, but I wasn't prepared for the phone call I received during Laura's senior year.

"Laura has been chosen to be part of the homecoming royalty," the voice said. "Don't tell her! We want to wake her in the morning, take her to breakfast and surprise her. The king and queen will be announced at the homecoming assembly next week."

The auditorium of Pine View High School was packed with students during the homecoming assembly. One by one, each elected member of the royalty was introduced and greeted with thundering applause. As Laura stepped onto the stage, the crowd went wild.

When Laura was crowned Homecoming Queen, the audience jumped to their feet in a standing ovation. Tears poured from my eyes. My heart was bursting with joy knowing that genuine caring and acceptance filled the room.

Laura was a beautiful queen who proudly represented her school. As she was presented to the audience at the football game, she waved and smiled sweetly to her fans from the back of a convertible. Once again the crowd rose to their feet. Many of the adults were touched and cheered through tear-filled eyes, but the students were just cheering for their friend.

Ben, the homecoming king, called her "The Queen of Queens" and gave her a bouquet of roses. Travis, a long-time friend, came home from college to take her to the dance the next night. She radiated such a spirit that all could feel the happiness in her heart.

I couldn't believe it. All the fears I once had were replaced with feelings of gratitude. I felt gratitude to God for blessing me through the years with knowledge of how to raise Laura and gratitude for her friends who so willingly included her in their activities.

Adele Tolley Wilson

Robin

One of my favorite things to do is sit on the front porch with Robin and wait for her school bus to arrive. We sing "The Wheels on the Bus" and other songs she loves. When the bus arrives she runs off, waving to me and yelling, "Bye, Mom."

As I watch her bus take her to 6th grade I often think back to twelve years ago when we found out I was pregnant with my eighth baby. Because she was developing slowly in the womb and because I was forty the doctor did an amniocentesis. We found out that she would be our eighth daughter and that she had Down syndrome.

We were fortunate to have a few months to prepare for her arrival so we visited with a genetics counselor, attended a support group and read what we could about children with Down syndrome.

Everyone loved and spoiled Robin and she was a delightful, sweet baby. We continued to attend the support group and had visits from a nurse who taught us what we should know and do during her infant years.

However, as much as I loved Robin, I was still angry and bitter because she wouldn't have the choices that her seven older sisters had. She probably would never drive a car, go on her first date, join the high school band or color guard, attend college, choose a profession, or marry and have a family of her own.

Why did Robin have to be different? Why would her life be a struggle for her and those around her? Would she understand when other children stared at her or made fun of her? Why would life have to be so hard for my sweet baby girl? So I prayed hard and often. I prayed not to change Robin, but for understanding and peace.

When Robin was a few months old and I was still wrestling with these feelings, I was driving home from work during rush hour and thinking about her. From out of nowhere came a voice, "She doesn't care."

"What?" I asked the voice in my mind.

"She doesn't care," the voice answered. "She knew who she would be before she came here and she doesn't mind, so why should you?"

Instantly the anger and bitterness left, replaced by peace and joy. I understood that Robin knew who she was and it didn't bother her, and from that moment it has never bothered me either. Life would still be a struggle, but isn't it for everyone? Life with Robin is an adventure and we're glad we're on it with her.

Karen Leeper

McKay

A s parents of seven children, my wife and I have experienced our share of minor medical challenges. Doctor's visits, visits to emergency rooms for stitches, and a couple of minor surgeries have been the norm. As a matter of fact, the only real medical challenges we had ever experienced were the deaths of our fathers and a mother's survival of a serious case of cancer.

We felt very comfortable that life was going smoothly and that our children's medical challenges wouldn't be any different than ones we experienced growing up. When we found out we were pregnant with our eighth child our sense of complacency lulled us to sleep. Our wake up call came when McKay was born. We immediately knew something was different. Something was special about this little boy who we knew had come to complete our family.

Because of heart problems McKay spent his first three weeks of life in the local children's hospital. As we made our trek each day from our home 45 miles away, my wife and I had time to ponder, reflect, and more importantly count our blessings that the challenges ahead were "manageable."

We had the opportunity, daily, to see first hand what other parents were experiencing. We saw children who wouldn't see their first birthday, children whose stay in the hospital would be ten times the length of McKay's, children whose lives would revolve around the hospital. We were grateful our son's stays in the hospital would be relatively short and few.

As McKay approached six months his doctors began to discuss with us the extensive surgical procedure that would provide a great measure of relief to the pressure his little heart was experiencing. We were told the procedure was common. Despite the reassurances of medical personnel and friends, as parents we couldn't help but be somewhat concerned.

In between work, travel, baseball, ballet, and church we worked hard to make sure that nothing we could control would delay the procedures. We did everything we could to prepare and minimize the effect of the extended stay at the hospital on the other children. My wife and I even spent extra time together to make sure each of us was okay.

In the three days before McKay's surgery the tension in our home was electrifying. All of our efforts to "minimize" and "normalize" appeared to be for naught. The children were more emotional than ever and the tension between my wife and I was accentuated by a teething baby, and a genuine fear of the unknown.

On the morning of the surgery, 5:00 a.m. seemed to come earlier than ever. As we loaded McKay into the car to drive to the hospital, my stomach in knots, I marveled at the stillness in the air. I wished somehow I could take a deep breath and fill myself with calm.

As we passed through the revolving doors into the hospital the sense of concern heightened. Each step toward the operating room seemed to increase the emotions. In the hour and a half we waited prior to surgery we prayed silently and together.

In the final minutes before walking McKay to the door and leaving him in the arms of the anesthesiologist we gave him a blessing. In that blessing we asked for comfort in knowing everything would be fine. Never in my life did I ever imagine how that sense of comfort would come.

As I passed my precious son to the anesthesiologist I took a deep breath trying desperately to drink in the calmness I had felt in the air earlier that morning. I reflected on the blessing given just minutes before. I heard audibly in my mind the many prayers that had been said in his behalf.

My eyes followed the anesthesiologist as he turned to walk down the hall to the operating room and I was immediately filled with calm. Standing on both sides of the anesthesiologist, with loving smiles and dressed in white, I saw McKay's grandfathers.

Stephen Meacham

Heidi

As I walked into Heidi's bedroom, I automatically went over to shut the blinds against the darkness that had engulfed the cold December air outside. Our cheerful green and red swags of holiday lights glistened in front of her big window. I let go of the strings and thought, "Tonight, I'm going to keep her blinds open so she can see the lights from her room."

How she loves the beautiful Christmas lights sparkling from our rooftop and trees. She is the one who makes sure that they are plugged in after school. I know it is a bit of a waste of electricity to have them running in the daylight, but it's one of the few joys she experiences, so I let it slide. There are some plugs outside that she can't reach, so the minute my husband, Rod, gets home she declares, "Dad, lights!" over and over until the job gets done.

She seems to enjoy going with me in the car in the late afternoon on errands. It's not so that she can pester me for gifts or treats in the stores. Mainly, I think it's so she can see the pretty decorated homes and yards around town.

When Heidi and I are out driving my mind is busy going over the hustle and bustle of this hectic season, so it's good to hear her occasionally murmur quietly from the back seat, "Christmas, Mom."

"Yes, Heidi, isn't it beautiful and wonderful?

She doesn't usually respond to me, but I know she knows that there is something very special about this time of year, and it reminds me to try to slow down and feel once again the childlike joy and wonder of it all.

It is music to our ears when she says anything. Through the years, our family has learned to always respond to even her slightest verbalizations in hopes of encouraging more communication from her.

It doesn't hardly seem possible that sixteen Christmas seasons ago, we were a happy little family at home enjoying our new baby, Heidi Ann. Her three older sisters, Torey, Lacey and Holly were thrilled with this tiny, sweet little newborn. Little did they know or even care what the words "Down syndrome" meant and that we would all be traveling a different path since Heidi had come in our lives.

Looking out Heidi's bedroom window at the falling snow, I loved the beautiful serenity, but mostly I felt exhaustion. After bathing Heidi, I flopped on the floor in her room and tried to prompt her to dry herself off and get ready for bed. She just sat there so I was very grateful when Rod stepped in with her lotion, diaper, and "jamies" and got her ready for the night. He was done and cheerfully slipped out humming the beautiful haunting

Christmas melody of "Greensleeves" and "What Child Is This?"

Her mood changed for the better, Heidi looked at me and a sweet expression lit up her face. She walked over and picked up a framed picture of Christ. Without saying a word, she brought it over for me to look at. I was touched by her unusual and thoughtful gesture.

"Oh, Heidi, thank you for showing me this," I responded softly. Then quite automatically, always trying to encourage more interaction I asked, "Who is this, Sweetie?"

Her eyes had a certain glow and expression that we only occasionally glimpse, "Jesus," she said softly, smiling.

"Yes, that's right, Heidi." Then hoping she somehow knew of His great love for children and especially those with physical and mental problems, I said, "Is Jesus your friend?"

She nodded her head in understanding. My eyes welled up with tears as I fondly recalled the previous December when a similar setting evolved in this room. I had set up a simple nativity scene in Heidi's bedroom for the holiday season. Again, she was drawn to the baby Jesus in the manger and picked it up.

I said, "Heidi, who have you got there?" No reply. "Who is that baby, Heidi?"

Her eyes sparkled and she replied warmly, "Jesus."

"Yes! Good talking, girl." Not wanting this opportunity to slip I curiously threw out another question, "Heidi, what can you tell me about baby Jesus?"

She thought for a second and said as plain as day, "The star."

I caught my breath and said, "The star of Bethlehem?"

"Yes," was her simple reply.

As I put the little manger piece back in place, I wondered if it was just too lucky to really be true. I had to test it again.

"Heidi," I asked hesitantly, "thank you so much for telling me that. What else do you know about Jesus?" I pulled her covers up around her shoulders. "Can you remember anything about Jesus?"

She paused again and looked steadily at me and said clearly, "The Son."

By this time I was softly crying, as I said, "The Son... of God? Is that what you mean, Heidi?"

"Yes," was her honest answer.

I knew that I had been given such a precious gift this night, but I was still so hungry for more. I knew Heidi was tired and wanting to roll over and sleep, but I pressed her for one more interchange. "Heidi, can you tell me anything else about Jesus?"

Somehow she knew I desired more spiritual insights to give me strength, as it had in the past. She paused and looked me right in the eyes and simply explained, "Church."

I nodded knowingly and said, "Thank you so much. Good night, Honey."

That was such a sweet and special memory to me, and it helped sustain me through some of the rough times that previous year. Sometimes I would ponder who and what child _is_ this?

I wondered if I was to ask her that same question tonight, what her response would be, or would there even be a response? I certainly knew her moods ran hot and cold, and I often doubted that she really remembered or even comprehended any of the Bible stories from church.

"Heidi," I said as I put back the Savior's picture, "can you tell me something about Jesus?"

She thought for quite a few seconds and her reply was the same as it was a year ago, "The star."

Again, it took my breath away and I asked, "Do you mean the _new_ star in the sky?"

She had an angelic look on her face and calmly said, "Yes."

Oh, how precious this was to me. I almost didn't dare continue for I was a little afraid this sweet and spiritual exchange would take a turn in another direction.

"Heidi,... Mommy wants to know _anything_ else about Him that you know. What do you know about Jesus Christ?"

I could tell by her expression and her searching eyes, that she was traveling in thought to a place that she had experienced long ago. For a few moments her eyes were gazing up in deep thought and then she turned.

"The King," was her simple reply. That was enough for me…enough to last a lifetime.

Elayne Ann Potter Pearson

Matt

Our son Matt was born April 11, 1977. I was 25 at the time, he was our second son. My husband had a very strong impression several months before he was born that our baby would have Down syndrome.

Having a son with Down syndrome was a big adjustment for me. But I found that every time I felt sad or depressed or frightened or uncertain, all I had to do was pick him up and hold him and I felt the most overpowering feeling of peace, love, and well-being.

Unfortunately, Matt had quite a severe heart defect. At age 5 we took him to Rochester Minnesota to the Mayo Clinic for open heart surgery. He lived four months and passed away February 11, 1983, just two months short of his 6th birthday.

More than 20 years have passed since he left us but it seems like it was yesterday. As hard as having him was, losing him was much, much harder. When he passed away, a very real, tangible light went out of our lives. It was just like someone dimmed all the lights and they've remained that way ever since.

We believe that families will be reunited after death. We look forward to the day when we can be with Matt again. I can't wait to get to know him.

Jeannie Workman

Kenly

People often ask, "Is she yours?" And why wouldn't they? With her long, blonde hair and sky-blue eyes, Kenly Marie doesn't look a thing like her dark-haired father or brown-haired, brown-eyed mother. Not to mention the Down syndrome, distinctly setting her apart from the rest of us. But yes, she is ours---biologically, emotionally, eternally, and in every other way.

I often wonder what events took place in Kenly's pre-existence to make her a part of our family, the part that would forever alter the way we look at life and its meaning. I like to picture her great-grandfather Theodore, a wonderful man who passed away six years before she was born, involved in a post-mortal conversation with his friend, Homer, who knew first-hand the joy of having his own blonde granddaughter with Down syndrome.

"Theodore," he says, "we must arrange for you to have a similar blessing for your own family. The joy she will bring to your loved ones and the lessons she will teach will be of great worth to your posterity."

In this daydream, everything is approved and arranged, and Kenly is sent to us. We deal with the initial grief and anguish and over time come to see that, yes, there is no other blessing quite like this one.

The blessing of having a child with special needs is not without its challenges, however. It is a time-consuming, high-stress job dealing with the delays, medical concerns, and constant care. When Kenly was younger, I often felt overwhelmed and worn-out. Time alone as a couple seemed non-existent.

In December 1998 when Kenly was three, my husband and I took a respite trip together, leaving our two little children in the care of their grandparents. It was a much-needed break but, as mothers do, I worried about leaving my children. I was especially concerned about the last night and morning of our absence when my brother Robby, who had never tended children, would be watching Kenly and our 9-month-old son alone.

We arrived home from the airport to find all was well. I wanted to ask Kenly how things had been, but with her tremendous speech delay this was pointless. She was barely saying "Mommy" and "Daddy." Instead, I pointed to my brother and asked, "Kenly, who was watching you while we were gone?"

Without hesitation, and as distinctly as I had yet heard her speak, she answered, "Theodore."

Yes, she is ours. But she is not ours alone. I do not know what transpired in Heaven to allow our sweet daughter to come to us, but I do believe that we are not alone in her upbringing. There are many family members who have gone before us who are anxious to see her succeed in mortality. I truly believe her special grandfather is even now a part of her life as she faces her challenges upon the earth. And he will be watching over her.

Amy Burton Moore

Jesse

I was afraid that my little boy Jesse would be limited by his having Down syndrome. Little did I know that Jesse would be limitless in what he could do. He is aware of life and if he sees something he wants to do, he goes for it without letting fear get in the way.

Once we went to an amusement park and Jesse saw a ride that went upside down. He wanted to ride it. I looked at my husband and said, "You go with him." My husband said, "No way!" So, I went on the ride with Jesse and wondered at his fearlessness.

Jesse is my superhero. He challenges me everyday to look at life differently.

Cory McName and Jerry McName

Peter

I never intended to become a teacher of children with Down syndrome. My journey to teaching began more than 35 years ago when I met a boy with a happy square-like smile and sparkling eyes. I was a college volunteer in Eau Claire, Wisconsin. Peter took my hand and led me to his favorite sitting area. He was probably 10 or 12 years old. We sat as he studied me. I remember thinking, "Will I pass?" After a small while his body began to rock. Then he stopped, took my hands, still with his smile of acceptance on his face and pulled and pushed my hands until my rocking was more than obvious. Laughter spilled out into the room contagiously. Other Down syndrome residents joined in and by the end I, too, was laughing with the moment.

Peter had captured me. We were friends. All the joys and sadness life would bring to us during our time together we would share.

One day Peter greeted me with only his hands. He was looking down. There was no smile, just a walk to his favorite sitting area. I asked why he was sad and the tears came. His friend was hurt. His compassion for another was as real as anyone could feel. He would shake his head, showing a sense of loss of how to help his friend, and rock. I tried to console him with tenderness but also realized he needed to act. So he and I came up with a plan. We went shopping. Peter took his money and bought a stuffed animal and then we went to visit his friend. The smile was back and so were the hugs for one another. After realizing he was with his friend he turned to me with his smile and my hug.

Years later, while traveling through Europe on a train, I met a Dutch woman who invited me into her home for several weeks. She was a teacher. Her classroom was for handicapped children. I automatically joined in with Peter's kin. I shared stories of Peter from America. What a delight to be a volunteer for two weeks in her classroom.

I remember it was Thursday and Thanksgiving. During the meal my Dutch friend told me to go back and finish my college education in Special Education. She liked how I taught and loved her students. And she also knew that Peter had really made an impact on my life. I agreed, with a few negotiations for her to come to see America after my completion of college. She came several years later and spent the summer, assisting me with my special students.

She smiled when I told her that I had decided to teach regular education with my Bachelors degree but something interfered. On Friday nights I would often walk through one of the college hallways en route to my studies and hear music. One Friday night

I decided to see what the music was all about. It was a special education dance. I watched free floating bodies move to a beat that became inviting, with smiles of familiar friends. I joined in. I guess one could say I crashed the party. After that, I joined in the dances often.

One evening a gentleman came up to me asked who I was and what I was doing there. I gave my reasons. He invited me to meet with him in the Special Education Department the following week. I went and received a scholarship for a Master's program in Special Education. After receiving my degree I taught more than 15 years.

My friends with Down syndrome have given as much to me as any friend I have. I'm always keenly aware of opportunities to enjoy these special friendships.

Dorothy Sackett

John

In our Church we have a children's meeting called Primary. Our Primary President wanted to let the other children know that our son John was just like them. One Sunday, she brought some cookies with her. There were different kinds displayed on a plate. There were chocolate, chocolate chip, peanut butter, coconut, raisin, and white cookies sprinkled with candies.

The President explained to the children that although these cookies looked different, they were all cookies. She proceeded to say that there are many children in the world that are different. Some have light skin, some have dark skin, some cannot walk, some cannot talk, and some run around like you and me. The differences do not matter to our Heavenly Father because we are all His children and He loves us very much.

The President then said, "We have a special person in our Primary and he can do some of the same things that each of you can do, like making his bed, and helping his mother with the dishes. Just like these cookies are different, this person may do things that are different from you, right? But, he still is a child of our Heavenly Father, right? Can someone tell me who this special person is?"

Then all of the children yelled, "John DeVore."

The Primary President said, "Is there something that you can name about John that is different from what you do?"

One little boy raised his hand and said, "John wears a zipper tie to Church. He doesn't have to tie it. He just puts it over his head and then zips it to his neck."

My heart was bursting with joy. I thought to myself, "If that is all that this little boy sees different with John, then that is okay."

Afterwards, the Primary children sang "I'll Walk with You." The first part of the song reads:

> If you don't walk as most people do,
> Some people walk away from you,
> but I won't! I won't!
> If you don't talk as most people do,
> Some people talk and laugh at you,
> but I won't! I won't!
> I'll walk with you,
> I'll talk with you,
> That's how I'll show my love for you…*

Linda and Doug DeVore

---

* Pearson, Carol Lynn. "I'll Walk with You." Children's Songbook. Salt Lake City: The Church of Jesus Christ of Latter-Day Saints, 1987. 140.

Janie

I feel I have a very bright shining star that has lived with me for 5 years. Her name is Marelane Jane Lane and she is 44 years old. We call her Janie.

Janie's mom, Lilie, and I were very close friends. We lived in the same neighborhood. I was called the neighbor babysitter and I took care of Janie when Lilie couldn't find anyone else. Lilie often had trouble finding someone to watch Janie.

Lilie and I stayed very good friends even after I got married and had children. Lilie's husband Marvin died of cancer in the early 1980's. Lilie and I made a pact that if something happened to me she would help raise my two kids and I promised her I would take care of Janie if anything happened to her. I just didn't think Lilie would die before Janie but she died of cancer five years ago.

Lilie died in October and I kept in contact with Greg, Janie's older brother. He was so stressed out and couldn't find anyone to help him with Janie. He was studying for a big test and he told me he just knew he wouldn't pass the test while he was worrying about Janie.

I started thinking about the promise I made Lilie. I called Greg and told him that if he didn't mind, I wanted Janie to come and live with me and my family. I thought Greg had fainted on me. Greg broke down and cried over the phone because he was so overwhelmed.

So many people tried to convince me not to take Janie because my kids were grown and I should do something else, but I had made up my mind.

I have to do everything for Janie because she can't do things for herself. I have to wash her hair, give her a bath, fix her supper, lay out her clothes and make sure she's happy.

My daughter has a child name Austin and he and Janie have been together for six years. The day he was born she held him in her arms. She loves babies. She and Austin are big buddies. Janie may not understand everything Austin says, but she always agrees with him.

Because Austin lives with me, he's around Aunt Janie all of the time. He has become a sensitive child and he respects other children with disabilities.

There are mornings I feel down and go get Janie out of bed. She laughs. When she goes to bed she's still laughing. That laughter and smiling makes my day better.

When I start up the steps to get Janie up my grandson will yell at me and tell me he will get her up. He opens up the door and will say, "Janie are you goin' to sleep all day? Well get up woman it's time to get up!"

Janie has so much love that it rubs off on people who really need it. I babysit for two two-year olds and I've watched both of them since they were two months old. If Janie is eating something and one of the girls wants a bite she will break what ever she has in half just to share it with the girls and my grandson.

Janie's a true angel. She brings sunshine to our family. I'm glad I made the decision to make her a part of my family.

Belinda Smith

Jeffrey

Our little 5-year-old, Jeffrey, is a happy, playful boy. He is smaller than most of the children his age and he doesn't yet talk. But, he has a way of finding a fan club wherever he goes. So we are not used to getting calls like the one we received recently from the father of a boy in Jeffrey's church class. The father said he wanted to bring his son, Sam, over to apologize to Jeffrey for being mean to him.

Sam had pinched Jeffrey and felt bad about it so he told his parents what he had done. Unfortunately, with sickness and the holidays we were unable to get the two boys together for a couple of weeks.

Our first Sunday back at church my husband, Joseph, took Jeffrey to his class. When Jeffrey saw Sam he acted scared and put his arm in front of his face. He didn't want to sit next to Sam. Even after a few weeks of being gone Jeffrey remembered that Sam had been mean to him. We were a little surprised by this.

That day after church Sam and his father came over to our house. They were sitting in their car for a long time. Sam was upset and shy about coming in. In an effort to make it a little easier for him, our younger son, David, and I invited them in for some cookies.

Once inside, Sam apologized to Jeffrey and Jeffrey signed "thank you." Then little Jeffrey gave a much larger Sam a hug. His head only came up to Sam's chest. This was a sign of love and complete forgiveness and we all knew it. Sam's demeanor changed instantly.

Sam, Jeffrey and David then shared the promised cookies. Sam soon realized that although Jeffrey didn't talk like him, he did talk with sign language. We shared how to say "cookie" and a few other words in American Sign Language.

Not only did Jeffrey gain a good friend from this experience, we too gained something invaluable. Our lives were touched by the magic of a small boy teaching us the power of forgiveness.

Melanie Miner

Austin

Motherhood has its challenges-some big, some small, and some unexpected. On October 31st, 1999, Austin Brigham Frampton was born. Little did we know from that moment on our lives would take a different journey.

I didn't see Austin for two days. I lay in one hospital, Austin in another. When I was released, my husband, Jason, and I drove an hour to the other hospital and not much was said. Depression and gloom filled my soul. Did I even want to see this baby with all the problems the doctor's had found? How could I possibly be the kind of mother this child deserved or needed?

As I entered the Newborn Intensive Care Unit for the first time, tiny beds lined the wall. Which child was my son?

The nurse said, "Mrs. Frampton he's right over there, the one with the pumpkin on the basinet. You can hold him if you'd like."

I wasn't sure how to pick him up without disturbing all the tubing. As I held our little Austin he looked so normal, surely the diagnosis was wrong.

Later that day the geneticists called us back and showed us Austin's chromosome sheets. The Down syndrome was confirmed. I sat there numb; I couldn't speak. Jason asked lots of questions and the doctor had all the answers, except the one's I wanted to hear. He said having a child with Down syndrome is just like having a baby die. The baby you wanted and thought you were having doesn't exist.

Jason was my rock; he assured me we could do this. Austin chose us. He had a purpose. Each day became a little better. Blessings were given, prayers were said, phone calls made. Little did I know what a precious gift we had been given.

Austin's eyes were filled with the peace of heaven and angels accompanied him. Everyone that held him would comment on his tangible spirit. I had a good friend that would come daily, sometimes twice a day, to get her "Austin fix."

My friend would say, "When I look into his eyes he knows so much. He speaks to me with such great knowledge. What does he know that we don't know? I have such a spiritual experience every time I am near him."

Surgeries were necessary to fix some of Austin's bowel problems. The most crucial surgery was at hand, and the doctors were not optimistic about the outcome. We flew the family up to Utah for a special fast. We met at the church in Oakley, Utah where our family knelt in prayer. Jason's father, who was serving a church mission in Africa, said the prayer. It was piped in over the phone into speakers for our family to hear. So many people, 60 to be exact, came together in our behalf. I felt humbled by their support.

We went back to Houston for the surgery. The doctor came out shaking his head in disbelief. He said, "He did great!" The five hour surgery had only taken two and a half hours and the news had been much better than projected. The first messy diaper in the hospital was a celebration like no other. We knew that the Lord had blessed us.

Our journey with Austin has made me a stronger person. Our family has more depth than before. People ask has it been hard? Of course it has been hard. But that is just life. We are so grateful to have Austin as a part of our family. He is true joy!

Shelley Frampton

Carolyn

Carolyn Anderson was walking at twelve months, potty-trained at age two, and reading simple words as a six-year-old – not bad for a child that doctors wanted to institutionalize. They had predicted she would never walk, talk or be out of diapers and had advised her parents not to waste much time trying.

Carolyn, the youngest of the Anderson's eight children, was born with Down syndrome in the mid-1960's. At the time, it was believed by many that children like Carolyn were uneducable. But Ruth Anderson, Carolyn's mother, was a stubborn and feisty woman who ignored the naysayers and spent hours exercising Carolyn's limbs and providing stimulation for her mind. As a result, Carolyn did learn and progress fairly normally for several years.

By the age of seven or eight, Carolyn could read simple passages, but her comprehension lagged behind other children her age. Her mind just couldn't grasp what it was she was reading. Carolyn, who had inherited her mother's stubbornness, was determined. For nearly ten years, she practiced daily and eventually learned to sound out some of the more difficult words. Still, she would read without understanding. Things weren't clicking.

For Carolyn, frustration was greatest when she tried to read God's word, which can be difficult at times even for those of us with normal mental capabilities. "I really wanted to read my scriptures," she explained, "and I knew that Heavenly Father wanted me to be able to read my scriptures. So I prayed and prayed really hard for Him to help me learn to read."

The year Carolyn was sixteen, Ruth's mother was hospitalized for an extended period. Ruth would travel to Ogden, Utah, to be with her mother at the hospital for two or three days, then drive the 200 miles home to be with her family for a day, and then return to her mother's bedside.

After an absence of several days, Ruth returned home to an excited Carolyn. "Go get your Bible, Carolyn," Ruth's husband urged. "Show your mom what you can do." Carolyn quickly disappeared and re-entered the room carrying her scriptures. She immediately plopped down on the couch next to her mother and began to read in a clear, strong voice.

Ruth, not wanting to appear too skeptical, turned to her daughter. "That's great, honey," she offered, "but can you tell me what it means?" Carolyn smiled, her eyes lit up, and she correctly explained what she had just read.

Ruth was astonished. After ten years of practice, something had changed...but what? Questioning Carolyn produced a very simple answer.

"Heavenly Father and His angels came, Mom. They taught me how to read. They changed me here," Carolyn said, pointing to her heart. "And now I can read. Heavenly Father wants me to be able to read my scriptures. He loves me."

Now, twenty years later, Carolyn reads simple novels and, of course, her scriptures, often with a dictionary at her side as she continually struggles to deepen her understanding.

Kelly Howell

Jeremiah

One month after my husband abandoned me, I found myself to be 18 weeks pregnant. That would be *very* pregnant in anyone's book! I was ecstatic! You see, years ago I was told I could never have children. So this miracle, however inconvenient, was welcomed to say the least.

The minute I found out I was having a boy, the Lord prompted me to name him. He told me to call him Jeremiah. And, so in utero, I talked to Jeremiah constantly. I read him scriptures every morning, and prayed with him throughout the day and during my evening prayers.

I went to Mary Kay functions, and had everyone say hello to my bulging stomach, by saying "Hi, Jeremiah." So, he was well known before he was born.

*   *   *

Before I formed you in the womb, I knew you. Before you were born, I set you apart. (Jeremiah 1:5)

*   *   *

The week Jeremiah arrived was a devastating one. I found out that he had Down syndrome, and he would need three open heart surgeries by the time he reached one year old. I cried a lot that week, not for me, but for my poor tiny baby who would endure things I'd never had to face: surgery, hospitalization, challenges in learning, growing, being different, being retarded, being handicapped.

After that week, my sister literally moved us from Chicago to Detroit with all we could carry. In one fell swoop, I went from being a professional woman with her own home to a single mother living with her parents. And as I sat on the back porch, on an unseasonably warm February day, I heard a still, small voice.

*   *   *

To whom much is given, much will be required. (Luke 12:48)

*   *   *

I felt the Lord was telling me that He specifically chose me for this awesome task, and that this special anointing was an act of trust. I felt so grateful, so undeserving, so blessed in that moment. Words cannot describe the peace that fell over my heart that day. It was a moment in time, when my spirit was awakened, and I knew that it was going to be a sweet, sweet journey to closeness with my Lord and Savior, Jesus Christ.

I soon found my church home. It was a small, unassuming church, with a pastor who seemed to direct all his sermons toward my inner thoughts. Rosedale Park Baptist Church was unlike any I had ever been to in my entire life, and I really didn't want to join it. It was too small, the choir too little, the church too tacky and obscure. Yet, the Lord called me to join one Sunday, and it has been the biggest blessing my son and I share.

It took months of classes to become a member, and at the end of these sessions, we had a little ice cream social. At that social, I told one person that Jeremiah was going in for his major heart surgery at the end of the week. From that one casual conversation, I received calls from various church members, but what astonished me most was the deacon who showed up in the surgical waiting room at 6:00 a.m. to help us pray. I had never known such support.

This initial visit was followed by daily visits from various church members for the next 25 days of Jeremiah's hospitalization in the Intensive Care Unit. After waiting 25 days for him to "come to" the surgeons decided that they'd better go in and rearrange things back to the original design. I called my new church on the morning before his third surgery and said I needed a baby dedication by 3:00 p.m. that day because this may be God's time to call Jeremiah home.

We had singing and praying and a dedication service in that little ICU room that day. And God was merciful. Seven days later we came home with a recovered baby. The surgeons pulled me aside, one by one, and told me it was my faith that had brought him through.

After the surgeries were over and our doctor visits had been reduced to twice a year I remember thinking that the rest of my children would be a breeze!

* * *

"For I know the plans I have for you, declares the Lord. Plans to prosper you and not to harm you. Plans to give you a future with hope." (Jeremiah 29:11)

* * *

As I continue on this journey, I learn so much from Jeremiah when I watch him in church, when I listen to his "sermons" as he paces up and down the living room floor, and when I see him humbly fold his hands each night to prepare for prayer.

He is special. He was chosen. He has risen above his infirmities to form a special bond between Christ and this family. I am still in awe that this stewardship was entrusted to me. I have no regrets, no remorse, nor was I ever plagued by feelings of "why me?" I knew from the start that Jeremiah was a special miracle, a special blessing, delivered from heaven in the cutest little package.

* * *

"...and the peace of God, which transcends all understanding, will guide your hearts and minds in Christ Jesus." (Phil 4:7)

* * *

Amen.

Carol Hill

Mackenzie

I believe we were given the ability to dream for a reason. Most people do not dream of having children that will not be like the rest of the babies, children and teenagers though. Most people never dream of a child being born with a handicap; mentally or physically. Well, I did, but at the time I didn't know it.

My wife, Jill, and I have been married 18 years. Three years ago times were not very good. We had two children, Erica, 15, and Tyler, 10. Our relationship was going down the tubes and we were attending marriage counseling. We had just sold our house and moved in with Jill's parents due to poor financial responsibility. Things could not get much worse. Then Jill found out she was pregnant. This did not help matters at all.

The whole pregnancy seemed unreal and I really couldn't get into the whole pregnancy atmosphere: baby clothes, furniture and baby toys. But then the due date was upon us. It was Friday night; I was in the operating room by Jill's head, and she was undergoing a C-section. The two doctors were busy trying to get the baby out. Finally, they were successful and pulled the baby up for me to see. I remember looking at her eyes and telling the doctors to send her back. There was no way she was ours; her eyes were slanted. But they just kept holding her up. Then I woke up and Jill was still by my side and pregnant.

Sunday morning we were on the way to the hospital. This was it. Jill was in labor for hours with no significant progress and the baby began to stress. We headed to the operating room for a C-section. I was by Jill's head talking to her as the two doctors began their procedure.

The doctors had a difficult time pulling the baby out. When she finally came they held her up for me to see. I looked only at her eyes. I thought I was dreaming again. They were slanted. I held her and looked again. I went to the crib and stared again in disbelief. I asked the doctors about it but they wouldn't say anything.

I then took our baby girl to Jill's side. I told Jill to look at her eyes. I hadn't told her about my dream so she had no idea what I was talking about. I told her again to look at her eyes; she thought I was trying to tell her she was blind. Then I told her I thought she was a Mongoloid (that was the only term I knew, I didn't even know the term Down syndrome). She began to cry and I tried not to.

Mackenzie spent the next four days in the Newborn Intensive Care Unit fighting to breathe and live. I kept thinking it would be better if she didn't make it. She would spend her whole life being poked and prodded by doctors, undergoing numerous tests, and being made fun of because she looked different. Fortunately she was a fighter, pulled through, and proved to me that I was only being selfish.

In the weeks after leaving the hospital, Jill spent every waking moment researching Down syndrome on the internet, reading every book she could find, talking to every parent she knew and attending every meeting regarding Down syndrome. She was becoming more and more depressed and stressed. I tried to tell her that she needed to let Mackenzie be herself, let her progress at her level and her pace just as our other two children did. They did not walk, talk or potty train at the same age.

Having two other children, we soon learned that we took what they accomplished for granted, especially the little things like sitting up on their own, crawling, walking and talking. After working with therapists and doing what we thought was right for Mackenzie I truly believe the best therapy was from her siblings playing with her. Playing was her therapy, she just didn't know it!

Mackenzie amazed and continues to amaze everyone she smiles at. Her siblings love her deeply and will go to the ends of the earth to care and watch out for her. She has brought Jill and me closer together. Mackenzie could not have turned out so wonderful without the both of us working together. I have learned the most important person I can communicate with, rely on and even cry to is my spouse.

Like I stated in the beginning, no parent really dreams or wishes that his child will be born with Down syndrome. But I know this, when I don't give up, when I work with my family and go with my parental instincts, the smile Mackenzie returns to me enables me to dream again.

Eric O'Bryan

Hannah and Sam

Glenn and I have six children together and two from our previous marriages...and then Sam. That makes nine – yes nine – children. No, we are not independently wealthy and do not have an extravagant lifestyle, but we do have a home filled with love, laughter and the joy that only children can bring into a home.

When I became pregnant with our eighth child, we knew that the pregnancy would be our last. It was a promise that we had made to each other, as each successive pregnancy was taking a toll on the physical limits of my body.

This last pregnancy was also fraught with a worry because I had high blood pressure and was being medicated. When my blood pressure reached a certain point, we could not avoid delivery any longer. At 27.3 weeks gestation I signed the papers to have a therapeutic induction performed. Three days later Hannah came, having passed away about 42 minutes before she was born, too little to survive.

A week later, after Hannah's burial, our daughter Rebekah asked if we could adopt a baby. Glenn and I were both a little surprised at her request.

Immediately, Glenn mouthed to me 'no'. So I said to Rebekah that I couldn't promise that we would adopt a baby, but I did promise we would think about it. Little did I know what the future would hold.

Glenn wanted nothing to do with welcoming another child into the family. His heart was still very raw, as was mine, but I felt so strongly that we were still meant to parent another child. I didn't know if it would be a baby or a toddler but I knew there was another member of our family still waiting to join us. Unfortunately, through more medical errors, we found out we would never be able to conceive another child of our own.

It took months for Glenn to finally agree to even speak with an adoption counselor, but he finally relented. He had prayed often during our pregnancy with Hannah and had been given a vision of giving a baby a name and blessing at the front of our chapel.

After asking in prayer why God had given him that vision if it wasn't going to happen, the thought came that Heavenly Father had never told Glenn that the baby in the vision was Hannah. As soon as Glenn got home, he told me about these thoughts and asked me to call Jean, a social worker, the next day.

Jean had placed many children with Down syndrome in loving families all over our area, so we knew she was the worker we wanted on our side. The interview was done in May, a home study was done and signed by September and we then began our wait.

After much discussion with our other children, we realized we had no due date to mark off, no growing belly to remind us daily that another child was going to join our family. Jake, then twelve years old, said that we all got to take turns growing our new baby in our hearts instead and that it would be much more fun to do it that way. So that was what we did.

We chose names for girls, for whatever reason believing that the only gender we would be offered would be a little girl. In November, our yellow Lab, Chance, gave birth to her first and only litter of puppies, so we were kept busy and hardly thought about our baby-to-come much at all.

That New Year's Day we decided for the first time ever to have our dinner meal at noon. At around 12:25 p.m. a toast was made to the new year, which was bringing a brand new baby to our friends (who had also lost a daughter) and hopefully to our family, too. This was something none of us would ever forget, as we would soon learn that at exactly 12:26 p.m., a very special little boy was born.

Four days later, Glenn drove our friends to the airport and I received a call from our social worker. A baby boy was born in northern Ontario and he had Down syndrome. The birth parents were not keeping this baby; they had already left the hospital and signed him off to them. Did we want this baby? I very quietly began to cry and said a simple "yes."

I had no idea what to do. First, I thought we would get a girl and now we had a boy. Second, I thought the baby would be much older. And third, no one was home to scream and dance around the room with! My heart was so overjoyed I was bursting. I emailed Glenn on his pager with a single line, "Congratulations my love, we have a 4-day-old baby boy." Glenn said he was looking at his lunch when he got that page. He couldn't eat; he just sat and cried.

I called the hospital daily to speak to our baby son's nurses, who constantly asked what his name was. I didn't have a name to give them, so I told them to think of one to use until we chose one. About a week later, we told them his name would be Samuel James. I thought I had lost the connection to the hospital because the nurse was in stunned silence. When I told them to pick a name they chose to call him Sammy. When I said his name was Samuel, she was shocked and said that Sam must really be ours.

I was beginning to fret terribly about the fact that Sam might not really feel like my child. Once I walked into the nursery, I went right to Sam's isolette. Through tears, I could see the banner the nurses at his old hospital had made for his arrival to our city taped up on the wall. They had sent all his old charts, lots of notes about how much cuddling Sam liked to do with his nurses and how much they would desperately miss him when he left.

When I first held Sam I couldn't bring myself to place him near my face. He was so absolutely beautiful, so incredibly perfect. He looked like our other children and I marveled at that miracle of life that was lying in my arms. Within a few minutes, I tenderly put Sam up to my face, terrified at what I would feel, or rather, what I wouldn't feel in my soul. With tears in my eyes and a trembling voice, I looked at Glenn and said "Oh Glenn, he fits."

Words cannot express my relief, my joy, my gratitude. Within minutes, the realization that for as much joy as we were experiencing, there were two other parents just beginning their lifetime of mourning miles away from us. How could I ever begin to thank them for giving me such joy?

Some people have asked us why we felt we needed to replace Hannah. Sam is not a replacement for her. In fact, the only peace I ever felt about Hannah's death was from something Rebekah said to me when Sam was only weeks old. We were in our van, driving back home from somewhere, and Rebekah, who was 8 at the time asked me if Hannah and Sam knew each other in heaven and if they had spoken to each other. I said yes. There was a little silence and then Rebekah said she knew why Hannah had left our family when she did. Curious, I asked her why. Rebekah said matter-of-factly that Hannah knew that Sam needed our family more than she did, and that after they spoke for a while, Hannah agreed to leave early so Sam could join our family.

From that moment, I have felt nothing but peace about losing Hannah. Sam's story must include Hannah, for without her, we never would have him. In Sam, we have the opportunity to slow down, to see life from a very different perspective and to learn the processes needed to accept everyone for whom and what they are yet to become, not what they seem to be or what other people judge them to be capable of. We've learned that we still cannot tell the future, but we can sure enjoy the trip getting there. And we've learned all this because of two very special children, who never fail to bring a tear to my eye, joy to my heart, a twinkle in my step and most of all, gratitude for the blessings that God has given to us.

Glenn and Joanne Wilkinson

Reed

A month or so before Reed was born, I made this statement to my husband, "Everyone is potty trained and mobile. I'm not baby hungry any more, our youngest is seven. What if I talk to the school district about teaching part-time this year? We can certainly use the extra money. I could even be home for lunch to feed the kids when they come home."

Then I added the kicker, which we should never say because that opens up the way for the Lord to stir things up in our lives. I said, "This is the perfect plan!"

Bob and the children thought that it was indeed the perfect plan. I hadn't taught Special Education for 17 years, so this seemed like a challenge, but everyone agreed to help.

In order to renew my teaching certification I had to take a class at Brigham Young University. The class was a workshop which lasted most of the day and went for a week. In the meantime, Bob went to California to a conference for his work.

When I came home on Monday afternoon my daughter Jill told me that someone from social services had called me. This made me curious, so I called the office. The social worker did not know me, and had to think for a moment about why he had called me. Then he said, "Oh, I remember, there has been a baby boy born with Down syndrome. Would you be interested in adopting him?"

Without a moments hesitation I said, "Yes."

The social worker told me that five other families were interested in this baby so he would put our name on the list. I remember thinking about that and marveling that times had changed. That six families (our family included) would be interested in a baby boy with Down syndrome touched my heart.

At that point in time we had five children, three of whom were adopted. Our social worker for those three children had retired, and because Bob and I were both over 40, we were no longer considered as prospective adoptive parents. Because of our advanced age our files had been closed, and we had not adopted for seven years.

When Bob called from California on Wednesday morning I told him we were being considered as adoptive parents for a baby boy with Down syndrome. He asked, "Do you remember how old you are? Do you remember that you are 42?"

I told him yes. He asked about teaching school and our plans about that. I could only reply, "Things will be okay."

We talked for a few more minutes, then he said, "I've got to get back into my meeting. Don't do anything! Let me think about it."

Bob went back into his meeting and sat next to a man whom he had met at a previous conference. As Bob sat down his friend, Steve, noticed him and asked, "What's the matter? You look like you are in shell shock."

Bob replied, "What would you do if you called home and your 42-year-old wife said, 'We have the chance to adopt another baby and he has Down syndrome.' What would you do?"

Steve was quiet for a moment, then said to Bob, "If you don't take that baby, I will. I will come to Utah and get that baby."

Bob couldn't believe what he was hearing. He looked at his friend, and then asked the big question, "Why?"

Steve replied, "A few years ago we had a baby girl with Down syndrome. She had a heart condition which couldn't be repaired. She died when she was three years old. If you don't take that baby I will."

On Thursday I went up to BYU and tried to concentrate on the class. At every break I went to the phones to call the office where the meeting was being held to determine which family would be chosen for this baby boy. I was told each time that everyone was still in a meeting.

Finally, near the end of the class I got up and went to the phones and called yet again. This time I was told that the decision had been made. The social worker said that we had been chosen as his family.

Reed came to our family on July 15th, 1983. That is the day that I was supposed to meet with the school district and sign a contract to teach school. When I realized this and thought of the events surrounding Reed's birth I felt that with God nothing is by accident and as I stand still and watch the unfolding of His wonders I see the blessings unfold.

Also, at this time I remembered my prayer for my children. I had been praying for a very long time that I could be a wise mother who would help her children grow up to be happy, obedient and unselfish. God sent Reed as an answer to my prayer. What a tender moment it was when I realized that.

I believe many times things happen in our lives that can help us see the hand of a loving Father in Heaven. I can now see in my own life ways He has given me opportunities to make so much more of my life than I could ever have imagined.

Karen Hahne

Stevie

When Steve wanted to show me affection, he quickly wrapped his arms around my head, roughly pulling my head towards his pudgy torso, cutting off my oxygen supply. I looked up at his squinty, blue eyes, pleading for my release, but he mischievously grinned with his prominent under bite and gritted his teeth, relishing his empowerment of my thin frame. Eventually, I pried him from my red face, flustered but never angered by his strength and humor.

Sunday School rarely turned into a doctrine-oriented class with Steve around. Most of the time I didn't even bother to open my scripture case. Many lessons are lost in my memory, and in their place reside *The Muppet Show* movie boxes on my lap, rancid burrito breath inches from my face, and grey Velcro's stroking my khakis. Despite these distractions, I thrived on the three hours I spent with Steven Lawson every week because he taught me the true significance of charity.

Steve only seems disruptive. As the intensity of the room augments, so does his seemingly endless stream of energy. Often this results in a conversation between his hands, his index fingers and thumbs joining together rapidly, speaking a fabulous language whose transcription would look like a page full of childish scribbles, a masterpiece of abstract art. These two, five-limbed minds can continually bicker, snicker and weep with each other for hours, and Steven's tremendous range of voices and sounds effects provide the medium in which the two communicate. Nobody knows what his hands are saying, but there's always the constant envy that they're having a much better time than the rest of the world.

In every Aaronic priesthood quorum meeting, Steve found that a bunch of immature young men provided the proper forum to entertain, to the dismay and delight of the teachers. Once, Steve pounded on the piano for half of an hour, deftly and powerfully avoiding the grip of our hypothetically authoritative teacher. Another time, Brother Hal Whitney asked that we ignore Steve's antics, but upon the outset of the lesson, Hal's mouth gaped and he let out a howl of hysteria as he watched a puppet show featuring Tigger and a faded baby doll from the nursery. Brother Gary Rolph integrated Steve's comedy into a tradition of questioning the Mexican-food-lover what he preferred on his burritos. The simple response made everyone smile. Steve rarely spoke discernible English.

"Salsa."

Steve never fails to inspire. During a church talent show, we granted him the opportunity to throw a pie in the bishop's face. To the delight of the audience, Steve did, faithfully believing that we would instruct him to do nothing but good. Seconds later, looking upon the abominable snowman before him and the spinning pie tin below, Steve allowed his short, stocky frame to droop with sorrow, either because the pie cream was spoiled or because he felt he had offended the bishop. My speculation was both. His joyful disposition soon returned upon discovering a smiling white face and some salvageable cream in the tin.

Steve shines. Brother Rolph was giving a lesson one Sunday on the importance of being a disciple. He rhetorically asked if we would stand as witnesses of Christ. When Steve quickly stood with a ridiculous smirk, all I could do was break into laughter. Only after glancing at the serious, enlightened face of Brother Rolph did I realize my spiritual ignorance.

At school, everyone was Steve's friend and wanted to pat him on the shoulder or shake his limp hand. His popularity became fully evident during our graduation ceremony as he received his diploma and waddled down the rickety staircase to a roar of screams, whistles and fog horns, undoubtedly the greatest cheer for any graduate. He responded by grasping the diploma and humbly raising it over his head, smiling with his usual splendor.

Steve is brilliant. He reads human emotion and spirituality like no one else. He intensifies feeling to the unfiltered, honest level upon which he operates.

His limited vocabulary has given him the wondrous gift of the language of the heart. Maybe that's what his hands are speaking.

This gift is most effective in Steve's dealings with the priesthood. He always recognizes the presence of the Spirit and wants to partake of its blessings. After class presidencies were set apart one Sunday, he hopped in the chair, hoping to feel the weight of hands on his soft hair. As a deacon, he passed the sacrament with understanding and grace. Steve's first Sunday blessing the sacrament brought me closer to Jesus Christ than I have ever been.

I almost immediately began to quiver as Steve slumped against the cushioned bench between Tyler Crisp and me. Although Steve's normally rough, dry hands were moist and extremely clean that day, we still had to wipe his hands with baby wipes. A terrible inadequacy consumed me as I gently washed the sinless hands. The opening hymn started, unfamiliar in my ears and on my tongue. It soon left me speechless and with tears in my eyes as I listened to its sweet words:

> For a wise and glorious purpose
> Though hast placed me here on earth
> And withheld the recollection
> Of my former friends and birth;
> Yet oft times a secrets something
> Whispered, "You're a stranger here,"
> And I felt that I had wandered

From a more exalted sphere.[*]

Although this poetic statement applied to everyone, that day it described the young man with Down syndrome sitting next to me. Steve's heavenly nature made him a stranger amidst all of the sin surrounding him on this earth. Still, he tried to perfect his acquaintances despite his physical imperfections with a love universal and timeless in nature. Indeed he had wandered to his mortal state knowing he would confront significant challenges, but also knowing he would return home to live with his Father. Steve is just trying to bring everyone with him. That's why he became my friend; he recognized I needed some extra help.

As we sat down from administering the sacrament, Steve wrapped his strong arm around my narrow shoulders and smiled. For the first time in my life, the Holy Ghost was tangible, enveloping me through the young man with pasty, rough skin, high-water pants and deep eyes next to me. Every aspect of Steve made the Atonement graspable and salvation attainable.

Leaving for college, I nearly missed an opportunity to thank my friend Steve. Luckily, I was able to visit his home before he had to get on the bus to his new school. Acknowledging the looming separation, Steve quietly said goodbye. I hugged his soft frame then left. Driving home I thought about

---

[*]Snow, Eliza. "O My Father." <u>Hymns of the Church of Jesus Christ of Latter-Day Saints</u>. Salt Lake City: The Church of Jesus Christ of Latter-Day Saints, 1998 ed. 292.

what Steve had taught me. Steve reminded me to constantly seek love and truth. To share all that we gain through service. To be like Jesus Christ. My lip began to quiver and my vision blurred. Thanks for reminding me, Stevie.

Luke Warnock

Postscript

I recently sat in a large room with hundreds of people whose lives had been and were still being touched by knowing someone with Down syndrome. We shared a common bond. There were hundreds of stories that could have been shared that day. The stories in this book are a small sampling of the many experiences of people touched by Down syndrome.

In an effort to encourage the continued sharing of stories about lives touched by Down syndrome a website has been established. Please visit www.ltbds.org to read more stories or to share your experiences with others. The goal is for this site to grow into a vast collection of stories that will uplift the spirit and bring many people joy as well as provide information for those who have just begun the journey of knowing someone with Down syndrome.